Herbal First Aid: Assembling a Natural First Aid Kit

Raleigh Briggs, 2005

Originally published in 2005

This edition © Microcosm Publishing, 2005-2022

ISBN 9781934620564

This is Microcosm #93

For a catalog, write or visit:

Microcosm Publishing

2752 N Williams Ave.

Portland, OR 97227

www.Microcosm.Pub

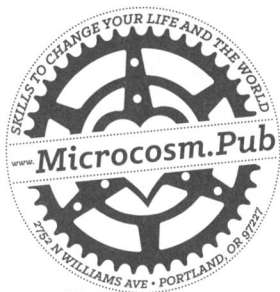

To join the ranks of high-class stores that feature Microcosm titles, talk to your rep: In the U.S. Como (Atlantic), Fujii (Midwest), Book Travelers West (Pacific), Turnaround in Europe, Manda/UTP in Canada, New South in Australia, and GPS in Asia, India, Africa, and South America. Sold to the gift market by Faire.

If you bought this on Amazon, we're so sorry because you could have gotten it cheaper and supported a small, independent publisher at Microcosm.Pub

Global labor conditions are bad, and our roots in industrial Cleveland in the 70s and 80s made us appreciate the need to treat workers right. Therefore, our books are MADE IN THE USA.

Hi! This is the companion zine to Herbal First Aid, a workshop i'm doing for DIY ACADEMY. most of the information in here was gleaned/swiped from the all-knowing, all-seeing internet. however, there are many good books out there on general herbalism and herbal healing. Here are two:

- The Herbal Medicine Chest
        by Douglas Schar

    This book has a lot of good information, including how to grow or wildcraft the herbs described. He also goes into (very Into) the chemicals that make plants medicinal.

- The Green Pharmacy
        by James A. Duke, PhD

    A totally exaustive resource about every single disease (almost) & how to treat it. This dude knows his stuff, and has some good stories about jungle rot.

    - Cat's Claw Herbal by Harmony

        This zine is totally adorable and really helpful. You can order it from MicrocosmPublishing.com

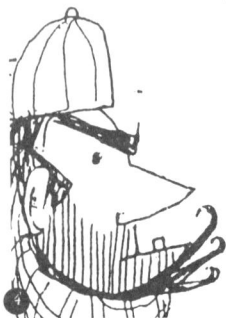

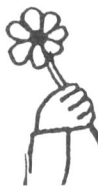

by raleigh b.
with drawings
by giovanni caputo

The KIT

First you need to take inventory of all your recent injuries and figure out what you need in your kit. For general kit, i would include stuff for:

- cuts + scrapes
- burns + contact rashes
- bug bites
- upset stomach + diarrhea
- headaches + muscle aches
- bleeding + bruises
- cramps + nausea
- random PAIN
- sunburn
- hangover!

- toothache
- parasites?
- zombies?!

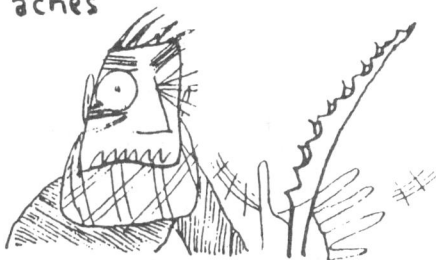

Second, get yrself a box, or a bag, or a tube, to keep all your stuff in. Or you can get a box and then a smaller box for a bike-sized first aid kit. Whatever you want.

Collect the boring, necessary stuff you usually keep in your kit. This includes:

- bandages
- surgical tape
- small scissors
- single-edge razor blade
- tweezers
- gauze
- rubber gloves
- eye cup/shot glass
- bandana
- maybe a small energy bar or bit of unperishable food

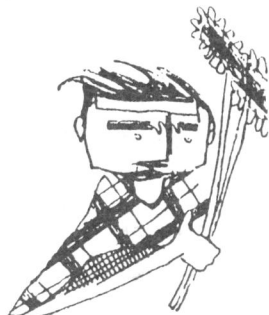

i come bearing herbs

Cuts + Scrapes

- Use cayenne, comfrey or yarrow as a styptic (to stop bleeding). You can keep a little bottle or baggie of cayenne that you can sprinkle on a cut. Yes, it does sting a bit.

- Dilute several drops of tea tree oil in a couple tablespoons of vegetable oil and apply to cuts, abrasions, fungal infections and skin irritations. Tea tree is a powerful antimicrobial, antibacterial, and antifungal agent.

- Keep an all-purpose healing salve to treat all sorts of mild cuts, scrapes + irritations. Tinctures are also good. Some herbs to use: comfrey, calendula, meadowsweet (as a painkiller), goldenseal, marshmallow, + horsebalm. Salves + tinctures can be found at co-ops and health food stores, but I've included directions to make both.

  To use salves: stop any bleeding with pressure directly on the wound, or by using a styptic. Clean the wound, then apply the salve. Cover with a bandage.

  To use tinctures: Stop bleeding and wash the wound, then either apply directly to the wound or pour on some gauze and use as a compress/wet dressing. Cover with a dry bandage.

  * Hey: this might seem obvious, but if your body reacts adversly to any of these remedies, stop.

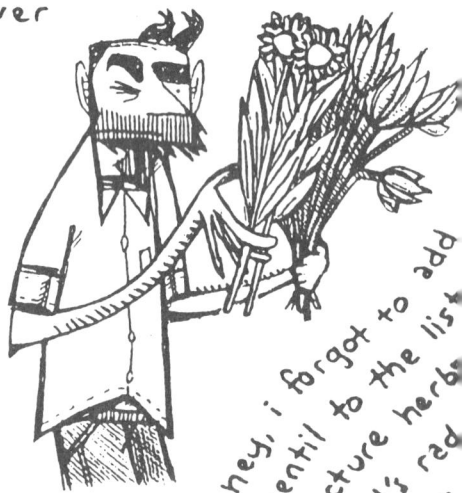

* hey, i forgot to add tormentil to the list of tincture herbs. tormentil's rad. sorry.

Gut Problems

• Keep ginger capsules or candied ginger on hand for when you feel nauseous, woozy, or have motion-sickness.

• If you eat something bad, try taking charcoal tablets (not the BBQ kind!) every four hours or as directed.

• blackberry leaf tea is good for the runs. Steep leaves for 10-30 minutes. If you have diarrhea, try eating cooked white rice, and make sure to drink a lot of water so you rehydrate. Raspberry leaf, slippery elm, and cranesbill can all be taken as tea to treat diarrhea. Yellow Dock tea is good for constipation.

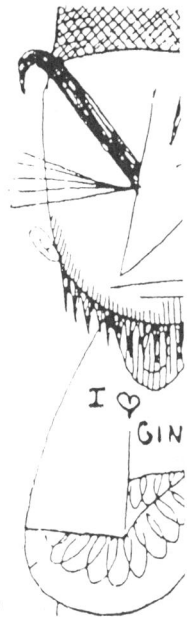

Aches + Pains

• A salve made with arnica, witch hazel, + St. John's wort will help cramped muscles — do not apply to broken skin. A massage oil made with your choice of oil plus essential oils of camphor, eucalyptus, rosemary clove bud will also work.

• Arnica tea can be used as a compress for sprains + dislocations. The herb will reduce pain, swelling + discoloration. Never use arnica on broken skin, tho Also, some people are sensitive to arnica, so stop treatment if you experience adverse effects.

• White willow bark (the original aspirin!), wild Let meadowsweet and valerian are all good anti-inflamm ory painkillers. Valerian is especially good for menstrual cramps— but be careful, you will feel a bit sedated. ❼

For headaches, stress, insomnia, & hangover, make an herbal eye pillow. Get yrself a square of nice soft fabric about 8 x 8", fold it so right sides are facing in, and sew along the long side and one short side (use a tight stitch!). Turn the pouch inside out and fill it with ½ -¾ c rice, ¼ c lavender flowers, and a few drops of lavender essential oil. If you don't fancy lavender, chamomile peppermint also work well. Stitch the remaining side closed. Any time you need to relax, lay back & let the pillow lay across your eyes.

Everyone should buy a bottle of Bach's Rescue Remedy. You don't DIY this one, but i still seriously recommend it. It's an incredibly soothing and safe formula you can take i all instances of stress or trauma.

Use oil of clove for toothaches (find this at the pharmacy). Put a little oil on a q-tip + hold it on the tooth.

• Rinse your mouth with a strong thyme tea or diluted tincture for a toothache, for sore throat or for wounds inside your mouth. Plain warmish salt water also helps sore throats + cleans wounds inside your mouth (or nose! Google "nasal irrigation").

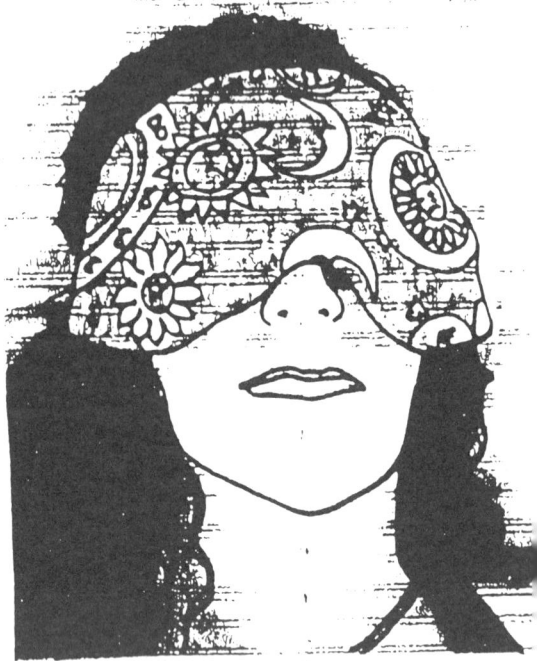

Burns + Rashes, plus Sunburn

✳ these remedies can be used for mild, small burns. Burns that cover large areas (even if mild) and burns caused by chemicals or electric shock merit professional attention. Moving on, then.

• Before you do anything else, hold your burned part(s) under a cold tap or bucket of ice water. Put an ice cube on a small burn. Cooling a burn numbs pain + prevents further injury.

• Don't put oil or anything oily on a burn. Oil retains heat + prevents air circulation + proper drainage, which slows healing.

• Some herbs that are good for burns are calendula, comfrey, chamomile, St. John's Wort, plantain + lavender. Tinctures will dry your burnt skin, so instead make a strong tea with the dried herb (say a couple teaspoons per cup boiling water) let it cool and apply as a compress. You can make this ahead of time + keep a bottle of it in your kit.

• Aloe, however, is the very best thing for burns. We all know this. You can purchase aloe gel, or make your own by puréeing together a cup of peeled aloe vera leaves with 150 IU Vitamin C powder (found at co-ops + pharmacies). The Vitamin C acts as a natural preservative. Store this in the fridge for extra relief. Combine aloe gel with any of the herbs above (in essential oil form), especially lavender!, for a really great burn salve.

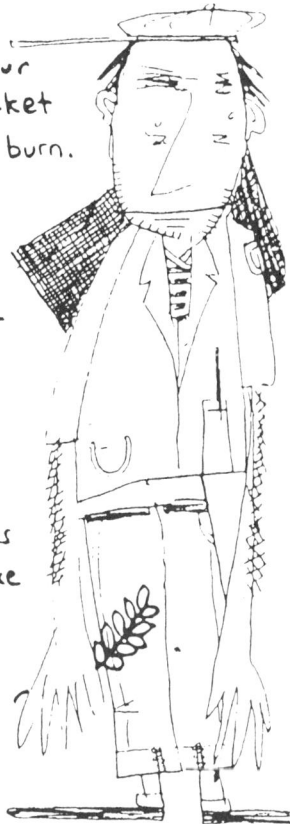

• For rashes, as well as almost any other skin irritation, calendula is awesome, as is marshmallow. Combine these tinctures with a natural, unscented hand cream for an easy salve.

• For Poison Oak + Poison Ivy, one website recommends a salve made **with** grindelia, echinacea, calendula, and white oat bark

• Make a poultice powder with equal parts gentian, ↗ buy in powder form or pulverize to dust in a coffee grinder myrrh gum, goldenseal, + marshmallow. Store in a ziplock bag + dust on sore feet, cuts (to stop bleeding), rashes, infections, and insect bites. Make a poultice for intense relief.

<u>To Use Poultices</u>: Combine powdered herbs with water to make a paste. If using fresh herbs, mash them into a pulp. Apply the poultice to the area + cover with a loose dressing.

<u>BUGS!</u>

• Make an insect prepellant by combining essential oils of lavender, citronella, eucalyptus, cedarwood, + lemongrass in a base of vegetable oil or equal parts water + vodka. Store in a spray or lotion bottle.

• Tinctures of witch hazel, plantain, grindelia, comfrey + St. John's wort are all good for itching. Lavender essential oil diluted in vegetable oil also works well.

• Make a bite-n-sting poultice by combining one tablespoon echinacea root tincture, 1 tablespoon distilled water, 1/8 teaspoon lavender essential oil, and 1 tablespoon bentonite clay. The paste should be tacky enough to adhere to the skin. You can make this ahead of time + store it in an airtight container. This poultice is really good for yellow jacket bites/stings + bee stings

Bruises + Bleeding ... plus Parasites!

• Once again, an arnica tea compress comes to the rescue. Other herbs that work well in tincture or tea form are chamomile, lavender, St. John's Wort or witch hazel. If yr at home, freeze some of the tea and place the tea ice cubes on the bruise.

• For nosebleeds, make a compress and soak it in one teaspoon yarrow tincture and one cup water, and place it firmly over the bridge of your nose. Lean forward + put your head between yr knees. You can also put another compress on the back of your neck and apply pressure to your upper lip. If bleeding is severe, try sniffing a tiny bit of powdered yarrow or agrimony. i haven't tried this before

• If you pick up an external parasite like lice or crabs, wash with a few drops of thyme essential oil in about 4 oz of water. I have heard that a slightly strong-er dilution of tea tree oil also works well.

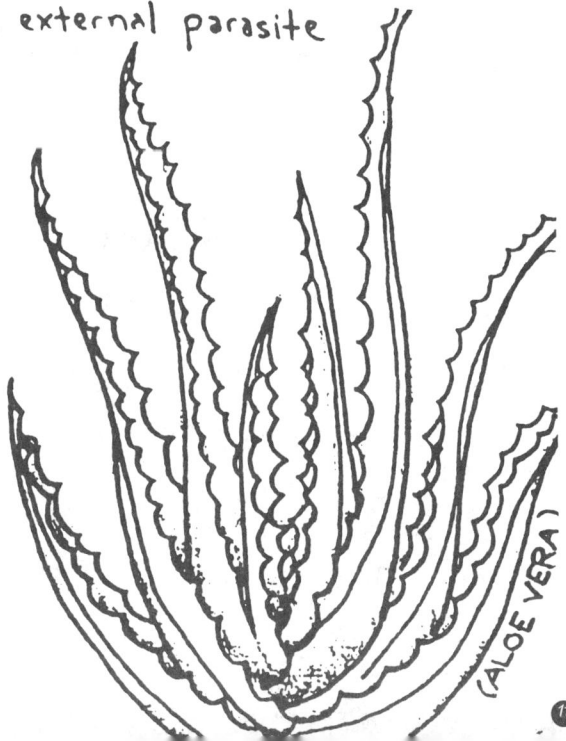

(ALOE VERA)

The How-to's

Making tinctures : Combine 1 cup chopped/ground dried herb and 5 cups cheap 60 proof vodka in a sealed container + let sit in a dark place for two weeks. Shake well from time to time. After two weeks, strain through a coffee filter and toss the solids. Store the liquid in dark glass bottles.

To Use : Tinctures can be poured on gauze for compresses, applied directly to a wound, or combined with creams or oils. To take internally, put 3-4 mL in a glass of water and drink 3 times a day or until relieved.

↗ sorry for the metrics!

Making Salves : On the stove, melt together 100 m olive oil, 25 g beeswax, and 25g anhydrous lanolin. In a separate pan, combine + warm 45 mL herb tincture of your choice, and 2g borax. With an egg beater, add tincture to the warm oil mixture, one drop at a time. Store in a dark glass or ceramic jar.

To Use : Apply topically.

Making Teas : Pour a cup of water (boiling, natch) over 2 T dried root and steep for ten minutes. Strain and drink.

Resources

- Jars & bottles can be found at co-ops, health food stores, and apothecarys.
  Borax can be found at the supermarket
- Candied ginger can be found in bulk at co-ops.
- beeswax + anhydrous lanolin you can get via mail order or in apothecary shops.
- Herbs can be bought, grown or wildcrafted. Look for bulk herbs in co-ops, specialty shops (like Travellers on Pine Street) or through mail order. If you wildcraft, always make sure you are totally sure what plant you have before you use it medicinally!

  Here are a couple places to get herbs:

- Mountain Rose Herbs (www.mountainroseherbs.com)
- Blessed Herbs (www.blessedherbs.com)
- Wild Roots (www.wildroots.com)
- Glenbrook Farms Herbs & Such
       (www.glenbrookfarm.com/herbs/)
  - www.oldtimeherbs.com

More from www.Microcosm.Pub

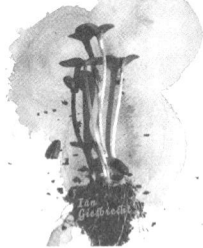

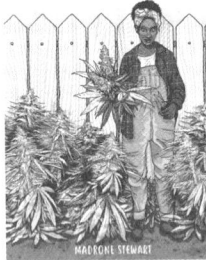

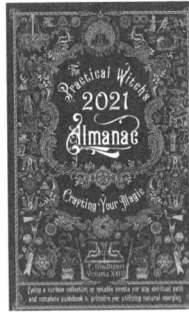

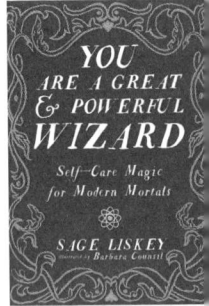

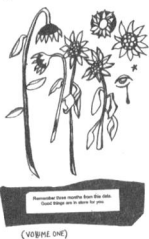

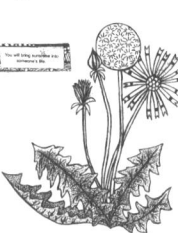

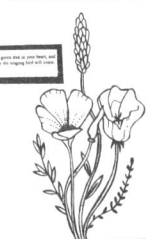

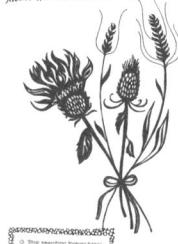

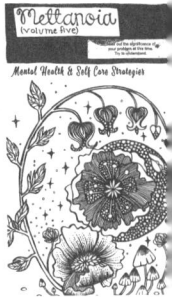

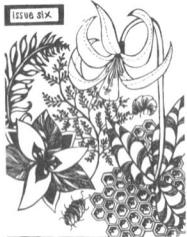

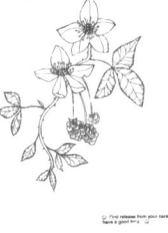

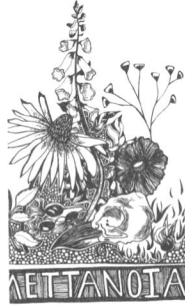

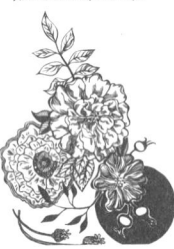

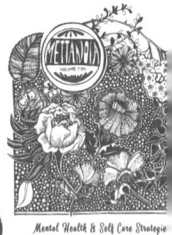

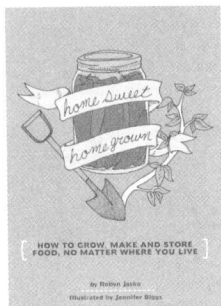

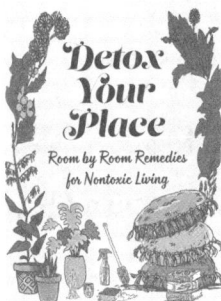

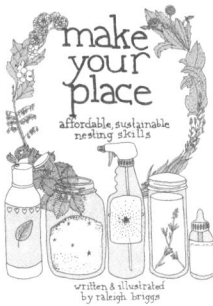

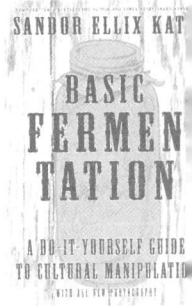